T0368700

Other books by Vivian D. Cate

Vegan Cuisine
The Proverbs 31 Woman's Resume

Also by Vivian D. Cate

Past staff writer for Firefighter EMS Journal
Edited Kids Evangelism Explosion teacher's manual
Wrote newsletters for Shepherd's Staff Ministries
Edits mystery suspense books by Laurie A. Perkins

INTRODUCTION TO HEALTHY LIVING:

Recipes for Life

VIVIAN CATE

WESTBOW
P R E S S®
A DIVISION OF THOMAS NELSON
& ZONDERVAN

WestBow Press books may be ordered through booksellers or by contacting:

WestBow Press
A Division of Thomas Nelson & Zondervan
1663 Liberty Drive
Bloomington, IN 47403
www.westbowpress.com
844-714-3454

Scripture quotations are taken from the Holy Bible, NEW
INTERNATIONAL VERSION®, NIV® Copyright © 1973, 1978, 1984,
2011 by Biblica, Inc.® Used by permission. All rights reserved worldwide.

ISBN: 979-8-3850-3848-0 (sc)

Library of Congress Control Number: 2024924889

Print information available on the last page.

WestBow Press rev. date: 12/04/2024

Contents

Dedication

This book is dedicated to Joan Graeff Tarbell, a home economics major who taught me well in her short 53 years. I owe her so much gratitude for the tools she gave me that have helped me through the mountains and valleys of life. I love you, Momma.

Acknowledgments

Thank You, Lord Jesus, son of God, for salvation. Thank You, Holy Spirit for empowering me to write. May others be encouraged (John 20:30-31).

I will continually be thankful for my husband of 40 years who believes in me. Because of him, this eaglet has flown ... from Paraguay to Estonia, from New York to California. God still amazes me at what He has enabled me to do. Author, speaker, Director of Nursery/Preschool for a national conference. Bob, you are the wind beneath my wings! I love you forever!

My sons, Nick and Ryan (wife Anna Marie), and my daughter Amanda challenge and teach me to be a better person, to love unconditionally. I love you ALL more than you'll ever know!

And praise God for wonderful friends like Martha Neville (who has prayed for me through 40 years of friendship), Phil and Laurie Perkins (who have not only been amazing friends but also edit all my books!) Now I have even more friends through Winchester First Baptist Church. Special appreciation to Donna Tant for editing this book, and Debbie DeBoard who serves me, prays for me, and encourages others to purchase my books! This church family loves us well. They have served us in so many ways, encouraged and taught us by example! We have the BEST church family ever!

Prologue

Introduction to Healthy Living: Recipes for Life was inspired by *Vegan Cuisine*, a book I published in 2014. Since that time, due to multiple illnesses, surgeries, hospitalizations, and near-death experiences in our family, my husband Bob and I have extended our research. How could we develop healthier ways to eat and live?

Health is not just *nutrition* (what we eat). It also involves *exercise* (from walking to lifting weights and/or playing sports), *rest* (taking breaks from busy schedules and getting adequate sleep), and, most importantly, *faith* (growing in a relationship with God, the father of Jesus Christ.) In addition, all these areas impact our mental/emotional status (moods and behaviors such as anger, anxiety, depression, joy, and love),

As Bob and I continued to grow in our Christian faith, in 2023 we moved and became part of the family and ministries of Winchester First Baptist Church. We work six hours a week managing a friend's yard and home (intense labor for folks in their 70's), and I attend a Zumba class several times a week at a local gym. While researching healthier nutrition, we have altered our diet significantly and come up with new recipes!

In this book, I review the importance of faith, exercise, rest, and nutrition as "recipes for life." Included are some dietary information, updated recipes, and wisdom from life experiences. Enjoy this unique and comprehensive approach to healthy living!

In The Beginning: Plant-Based Diet

Did you ever wonder why, in the beginning when God created the earth, people only ate plants? God said *"I give you every seed-bearing plant on the face of the whole earth and every tree that has fruit with seed in it. They will be yours for food." (Genesis 1:29-30 NIV)* God created all types of animals, but, according to scripture, none were killed until Adam and Eve sinned. At that point, an animal was killed to clothe them. Later animals were used as a blood sacrifice for sin.

If we do eat animals, the Bible later provides instruction regarding clean and unclean animals, what we should and should not eat. We are told to only eat animals with divided hooves AND that chew the cud. *"And the pig, though it has a divided hoof, does not chew the cud; it is unclean for you. You must not eat their meat or touch their carcasses; they are unclean for you." (Leviticus 11:7-8)*

Furthermore, the Bible says: *"But all creatures in the seas or streams that do not have fins and scales --whether among all the swarming things or among all the other living creatures in the water -- you are to regard as unclean. And since you are to regard them as unclean, you must not eat their meat; you must regard their carcasses as unclean." (Leviticus 11:10)*

But why? Shellfish and pigs are scavengers. They eat garbage. Think about the toxins, decayed foods, and mercury, that go into our bodies when we eat pork, ham, shrimp, crab, and so on.

Another beginning … about twelve years ago, my husband walked into our local Whole Foods store and noticed a movie playing in the education center. "Forks Over Knives" was a very convincing documentary backed by research. Their goal was to empower people to live healthier lives by eliminating animal products from their diets.

Bob and I began reading books like *THE CHINA STUDY* by T. Colin Campbell, *WHAT THE BIBLE SAYS ABOUT HEALTHY LIVING* by Rex Russell, MD, and *THE ENGINE 2 DIET* (*The Texas Firefighter's 28-Day Save-Your-Life Plan that Lowers Cholesterol and Burns Away the Pounds*) by Rip Esselstyn. In 2014, we attended a class with food samples and met Rip in person. We were sold. Everything confirmed our decision to change to a plant-based diet.

Some folks were stunned and asked, "What do you eat? Salads? How do you get enough protein?" Rip Esselstyn's book made our change quite easy by providing clear information and delicious protein-rich recipes. He even dispelled common myths, backed by scientific facts, about eating a plant-strong diet. As a firefighter in Austin, Texas, reportedly 70% of their calls were not fire related but medical emergencies. He saw firsthand the need for Americans to change to a healthier diet. I strongly recommend you get his book. The first half provides facts and information along with his own story plus the changes his coworkers experienced as they changed to a plant-strong diet. The second half provides all kinds of delicious recipes to help you make the change.

Soon, we began to explore and came up with our own recipes. Dairy free ice cream, entrees with beans or plant-based meatless products, taco soup, eggplant spaghetti, key lime chia pie, and so much more. As a result, in 2014 I published my first book, *Vegan Cuisine*.

Did we see the results? Bob lost 50 pounds to my 30-pound loss. My health improved as well. For ten to fifteen years, neither of us was sick (despite my history of pneumonia or other respiratory infections every spring and fall). A nurse practitioner coworker at the time also reported losing quite a bit of weight after changing to a vegan diet. She noted that her triglycerides dropped from 501 to 194 and LDLs from 128 to 88.

Many of the benefits of a plant-based diet are less visible. Reportedly there is less plaque in arteries, lower cholesterol levels, and less risk of cancer, heart disease, and diabetes. In fact, some diseases were reversed when people made this dietary change.

A Scientific Perspective

Scientifically, meat has no fiber which helps move food through the digestive system and prevents constipation. Furthermore, meat has no phytonutrients while vegetables, beans (legumes), fruits, seeds and nuts are healthy sources of phytonutrients necessary for health and prevention of diseases. Thirdly, much of our meat is contaminated by antibiotics, steroids, and so on. Notice how huge some chickens are in the store versus how they appear in a neighbor's chicken coop?

In "Forks Over Knives" T. Colin Campbell, PhD and Caldwell Esselstyn, Jr. MD use their scientific and medical research to provide convincing insights into adopting a whole food, plant-based diet. They believe that modern day diseases can often be prevented, halted, or even reversed by eliminating animal based and highly refined foods from our palates.

Once again, Bob and I did our own research. Every fruit and vegetable that we looked up has a measure of protein (except for lemons). By reading labels and googling the nutritional value of various foods, we learned more about the presence of vitamins and minerals.

Buyer Beware: One of the cautions of a plant-based

diet (or any diet for that matter) is swapping dairy and meat for refined and processed foods. Just because an item is labeled "plant-based" does not mean it is without potentially harmful chemicals. Ideally, prepare your **own** meat-free, dairy-free recipes, using local farm raised vegetables.

Congestive Heart Failure

Several years ago, Bob developed a severe case of Congestive Heart Failure. By that time, we had "fallen off the wagon" and started eating meat a few times a week. Bob had gained back 85 pounds and was having trouble breathing at night (twenty to thirty second periods of apnea plus snoring that could wake a farmyard of animals).

We ended up in ER where, for 8 hours, I watched his heart monitor depict what seemed like every kind of cardiac irregularity there is. As a nurse, I was frozen with fear and concern. The doctors started him on new heart medications … and made plans for surgery.

I continued to pray and worry about the installation of a pacemaker to stabilize his heart. We met with the hospital dietician about a cardiac diet. She explained that if you divide a plate into four quarters, one fourth should be starchy foods (macaroni and cheese, spaghetti noodles, rice, squash, corn, breads), one half should primarily be vegetables with some fruit, while only one fourth should be meat and protein. She also put Bob on a 2000 calorie/2000 sodium diet. Bob stuck to this regime for many months and lost weight. Meanwhile, Bob returned to exploring the internet, learning more about healthy diets.

High Nutrient Diet

3 Steps to Incredible Health was the first book to capture Bob's attention after his bout with congestive heart failure and eventual installation of a pacemaker. Dr. Joel Fuhrman has written multiple books on healthy foods and meals. He expresses deep concern for the diseases and obesity of Americans.

In this book, Dr. Fuhrman discusses the importance of a high-nutrient (or high-density) diet to prevent diseases and aid in weight loss. He reports that, at the time his book was published in 2011, a medical study confirmed that his nutritional program was more effective than any weight loss program documented thus far in medical history. Not only does a high-nutrient diet help with weight loss but it also helps keep weight off.

The average American diet is full of low-nutrient foods that increase food cravings and lend itself to overconsumption. Dr. Fuhrman lists "allergies, asthma, acne, headaches, high blood pressure, diabetes, reflux esophagitis, lupus, kidney insufficiency, angina, cardiomyopathy, and multiple sclerosis" because of such diets (see page vi of introduction to his book).

A high-nutrient diet not only helps with weight

loss but can also reduce blood pressure and blood sugar levels. Please consult with your primary care physician as you make dietary changes. Do not change medication without your doctor's approval. In fact, if possible, keep a daily record of weight, blood pressure, symptoms such as headaches, vertigo or faintness, and report them to your doctor.

So, what constitutes a high-nutrient diet? Dr. Fuhrman has a list in his book (pages 4 and 5). On a scale of one to one hundred, greens are the highest with mustard greens, kale, turnip and collard greens ranking 100. Other high-density foods are spinach, brussels sprouts, cabbage, arugula, and Bok choy. Onions, asparagus, mushrooms, and carrots are also moderately ranked. However, 85% lean ground beef is listed at *minus* four with salmon, chicken breasts, eggs, whole wheat bread, pasta, and skim milk rated *below two*.

One of the benefits of *3 Steps to Incredible Health* is the guidance given by Dr. Fuhrman on how to transition to this new diet plus over 150 recipes to get you started. For your health and well-being, Bob and I highly recommend you get a copy of Dr. Fuhrman's book

Lectins and More

As we aged, I began having digestive or gut problems, Then, in early 2024, Bob was hospitalized for a week with profuse GI (gastrointestinal) bleeding. I knew we were in trouble when, loading him onto the ambulance gurney, he turned white as a sheet, eyes rolled back, and he slumped (I begged God not to take him yet). By God's grace, Bob made it through that hospitalization.

Meanwhile, Bob had begun reading *The Longevity Paradox* by Dr. Steven Gundry, a cardiologist, medical researcher, former cardiothoracic surgeon, and author. Dr. Gundry's extensive research on lectins (proteins in plants that protect them) revealed that lectins combine with carbohydrates and cause gut problems, inflammation, and even weight gain in humans. Because of his research, we started making changes to a lectin free diet. Bob even purchased an electric pressure cooker so I could prepare beans. (Note: pressure cooking destroys lectins rendering the food safer to eat.)

Dr.Gundry provides lists (page 225 to 233) of what he calls "Longevity-Promoting Acceptable Foods" as well as "Disease-Promoting, Life-Shortening Foods to Avoid." Among those to avoid are pasta, white potatoes, milk, bread, wheat, rice, quinoa, peas, green beans, soy, several seeds and nuts, cucumbers, tomatoes, squashes of any kind, bell peppers, oats, corn, and more.

I hear you groaning! Then what *can* we eat? There are many foods on the "yes" list… including dark chocolate! Broccoli, brussels sprouts, cauliflower, cabbage, avocados and seasonal fruit, greens, onions, carrots, and asparagus as well as breads made with cassava, coconut, and almond flour are also listed. Sweet potatoes and mushrooms are among the higher nutrient foods, and pressure-cooked legumes are acceptable on Dr. Gundry's lectin-free diet.

In her online article "6 Foods That are High in Lectins," Alexandra Rowles, RD (article updated on February 8, 2023) agrees that eating large amounts of certain types of lectins can damage the gut walls. However, cooking, sprouting, and fermenting foods can greatly reduce the lectin content of foods and make them safe to eat. For instance, eating raw or undercooked red beans can cause severe nausea, vomiting, and/or diarrhea. Rowles reports that "red kidney beans contain 20,000–70,000 hau. Once they're thoroughly cooked, they contain only 200–400 hau, which is considered a safe level (4Trusted Source)." When cooked, red beans are actually very healthy due to their nutritional value.

In *The Longevity Paradox*, Dr. Gundry also includes information on health issues such as weight loss and the effects of various foods on the brain. Reportedly phthalates, found in grains, beef, pork, chicken, and milk products, have been linked to endocrine disruption. This ultimately can block the real thyroid hormone from delivering its message. The result is that, even with a normal thyroid level, people can have symptoms (such as weight gain) of hypothyroidism. Therefore, Dr. Gundry suggests these products be avoided.

Like Dr. Fuhrman, Dr. Gundry also encourages eating greens. He says that one serving of leafy green vegetables a day can slow the aging process of the brain. In addition, due to a four-year study in Spain, Dr. Gundy endorses eating walnuts and drinking nine to ten tablespoons of olive oil a day to improve memory and cognitive function.

Further research reveals nutrients that support brain health include Vitamin B, Vitamin E, Omega-3, and choline antioxidants (consider turmeric, nuts, fish, eggs, blueberries, green tea, and green vegetables). Of course, in addition to diet, brain health can be affected by sleep, socialization, nicotine and alcohol consumption.

Because of our age, history of depression, anxiety, PTSD and panic attacks and other family history of mental illness, I dove into more research. Turmeric contains curcumin which may help increase dopamine and serotonin and help with memory. Sardines and salmon are excellent sources of Omega-3 (adding flaxseed to foods is a plant-based option). Note that low Omega-3 intake can lead to depression, mental decline, and mood disorders.

While eggs are not included in a plant-based diet, they are superfoods for the brain as they contain Vitamin B6, B12, and choline which regulates mood and memory by generating neurotransmitters, maintaining chemical balance to the brain, and potentially reducing the effects of aging on the brain. On the other hand, leafy greens provide minerals, vitamins, and flavonoids which support immunity, health, stress levels, and fight age-related brain diseases.

Meanwhile, onions are highly recommended in your diet. Sources like WebMD report that onions are rich in chemicals that can lower risk of some cancers, protect your heart, and make it easier for the body to make insulin. Onions are said to be one of the best sources of quercetin which helps improve immune function and cellular health. Onions are also a source of fiber, vitamins, and minerals important for our health.

Shitake mushrooms add a meaty texture to soups, salads, and casseroles while providing Omega-3 and 6 plus 33% of the daily recommended amount of iron. They provide selenium, copper, potassium, magnesium, Vitamin B6, natural enzymes, Vitamin B12, fiber, Vitamin D. Lion's Mane mushrooms provide protein, iron, potassium and can boost cognitive function and improve nerve regeneration with possible benefits to those with dementia, Parkinson's, seizures, anxiety, depression, multiple sclerosis, muscle cramps. Big Mountain provides Lion's Mane Mushroom Crumbles which can replace meat in recipes. Meanwhile, our local supplier, "Fungalicious", grows and dehydrates a variety of mushrooms. They also accept mail orders (see Resource page).

Recently, hearing that Americans are often magnesium deficient, I did a google search. Magnesium is important for muscle contractions and heart blood sugar levels. Salmon, bananas, black beans, spinach, kidney beans, almonds and dark chocolate are good sources of magnesium.

When dealing with Bob's congestive heart failure,

I learned pineapples, cumin, and the skin of lemons reportedly help with edema. Grate several lemons and freeze for last minute seasoning. Lemon zest is delicious in casseroles and salads.

Prior to Bob's hospitalization for GI bleed, I explored the topic of fiber. Fiber helps support health and prevent several diseases. It helps digested food pass through the GI system. For an item to be considered high fiber it must have 5 gm. Some plant-based options include one cup of pinto beans, collard greens, carrots, cauliflower, prunes, seaweed, apples, black beans, lentils, pears, or avocado.

Unfortunately, wheat has lectins, so breads made of almond, cassava, and coconut flour are recommended. Sourdough breads are also acceptable as the fermentation process apparently removes or lessons lectins. Instead of oatmeal or rice, we use millet for breakfast (see recipes) or in place of rice in casseroles. For wheat free dry cereal, "Lovebird" has four varieties along with "Magic Spoon" (both can be found at Sprouts, Lovebird can be purchased at Whole Foods). There are also several choices for cassava or almond based pasta. We prefer Palmini angel hair noodles, made from hearts of palm.

Stevia replaces sugar in most recipes. While packages instruct using equal amounts of Stevia for sugar, we end up needing at least twice as much Stevia as we would need if using sugar.

Meanwhile, Omega 3 foods are important for heart, bone and joints, brain health or cognitive function, maintenance of healthy cholesterol, and for its anti-inflammatory properties. Men need 1600 mg. to women's 1100 mg of Omega 3. Some foods that contain significant amounts of omega 3 are kidney beans (406 mg/serving), pasteurized eggs (330mg each), walnuts (2570 mg/ounce), spinach (352 mg/1 cup cooked), salmon (2150 mg/serving), and flaxseed powder (2350 mg/1 tablespoon.) Keep flaxseed powder in the refrigerator and add to scrambled eggs, millet, casseroles, and so on.

Importance of Physical Exercise

Nutrition is not the only way to a healthier life. Physical exercise affects our muscles and spinal structure, the heart, lungs, gastric system, our moods, and so on. When anxiety reaches a peak, a good run has helped one of our loved ones. When depressed or anxious about life, a vigorous workout excavates (digs deep and removes) my stress, calms me, and enables me to refocus on the positive.

Exercise comes in many shapes and forms. I sit with an 83-year-old lady. After dinner we have music therapy, a sing-along session with friends around the piano. Then we go for long walks (she calls it "cising"!) Many retirement centers, nursing home facilities, and even gyms also provide opportunities for chair exercise.

Working with a group of women works best for me. If there is no accountability, I tend to slack off. Our gym, Mass Appeal in Winchester, Tennessee, offers a variety of group options such as Cardio/Stretch/Classic/Fit for Senior Citizens, Yoga, Pilates, Tai-chi, and Pump. Our church also has a small exercise room with weights and treadmills. Check out your options.

Recently I joined the gym and started attending a very high paced energetic dance class known as Zumba,

Wow! I could use my age as an excuse not to go back but I'm a spring chicken compared to a few other class members! In the long run, I appreciate the effort. It's such an invigorating way to start the day plus good fellowship.

One of my sons prefers heavy weightlifting to build and strengthen his body. He incorporates different machines and weights to zero in on specific muscle groups. My other son rides horses and works on the farm. One friend shared that, when she was growing up, she had severe breathing problems that required medications such as inhalers. When she was 31 years old, she decided to see if exercise would make a difference. Today, at 74 years old, she attends Zumba and other classes almost daily and has not had to use medications or inhalers since that time.

Studies have shown that there is a direct correlation between having more muscle mass and being able to survive chronic illnesses. Everyone should include some form of exercise in their daily routine. Whatever you choose, find a form of exercise that fits your age and abilities, and that strengthens you mentally and physically.

Rest and Sleep

It is equally important to balance diet and exercise with periods of rest and a good night's sleep. Sleep can help reduce chances of serious health problems like heart disease and it repairs your brain. Some sources say it even helps with inflammation.

Sleep not only helps physical health but it also affects mood and mental status. A person tends to think more clearly after an adequate night's sleep. It can also help reduce stress and minimize depression. Periods of rest during the day help rejuvenate a person who has a hectic schedule or intense load of physical and/or mental responsibility. Inadequate amounts of sleep can lead to poor quality of life, bad attitudes and difficulty with relationships, and can even jeopardize safety.

So how can we prevent these negative issues? Avoid technology before bedtime. Technology "wires my brain" and prevents me from going to sleep. Research supports this. Turn off TV, computers, and other technology two hours before retiring to bed. Avoid snacks after 4pm and eliminate caffeine and alcohol after lunch. Make sure your bed is comfortable, your room dark, and the house quiet. We use an air purifier (our "noise maker") at night to cover up snoring and outside noises.

Attitudes, moods, cognitive function, general health and well-being are improved with rest and sleep.

Healthy Body, Healthy Souls

The Bible describes our bodies as temples of the Holy Spirit. While it is vital to feed our bodies with healthy foods, get plenty of sleep, and to participate in some form of daily exercise, it is especially important to fill our souls with food that spiritually nurtures, strengthens, and guides us.

My life, like many of yours, has been a series of mountains and valleys. Sometimes those valleys have been horribly dark and frightening. Often, I have felt overwhelmed, alone, and abandoned. The Bible tells us that we *will* go through such trials. God even says He will never give us more than we can handle but will provide a way of escape. That way of escape is God. He is our safe place. *"He is my refuge and my fortress, my God, in whom I trust." (Psalm 91:2 NIV)*

God is my best friend. I share everything with Him, my joys and my concerns. He listens, He advises, He understands, He loves, and sometimes he appears silent. However, He is always there. If you have never experienced a relationship with God the Father, I would like to share with you how that can happen.

First, God is holy. He cannot tolerate or even look

upon sin. He is the Creator of the earth and everything in it. *"In the beginning, God created the heavens and the earth."* *(Genesis 1:1 NIV)*

God **spoke** ... and there was light and darkness, water and sky, dry land and seas, vegetation, fruit trees, sun and moon, fish, birds, and land animals. He is so powerful and almighty that all He had to do was **speak.** And then He created Adam and Eve. *"God created mankind in his own image ... male and female He created them."* *(Genesis 1:27 NIV)*

But, as our Father, God set boundaries. He had one rule. Don't eat from one specific tree. Adam and Eve had everything they could ever ask for ... food, friendship with Father God, a wonder-filled life ... but they disobeyed that one rule and sin came into the world. Therefore, ALL of us are sinners. *"For all have sinned and fall short of the glory of God."* *(Romans 3:23 NIV)*

Not only does sin separate us from God, but it leads to lawlessness, chaos, hatred, murder, abuse, addiction, and ... sin leads to destruction. God knew that, so He had to put a stop to sin. *"The wages of sin is death."* *(Romans 6:23a NIV)*

The only thing that can truly satisfy us is a relationship with the Creator. God wanted to restore that fellowship between man and God, so He sent His best, His son Jesus, to live among us as God yet as man. Jesus Christ lived a perfect life, unlike anyone else has or will ever be able to do. He spent three years teaching us how to live God's way, a way of love and self-sacrifice, generously caring for one another and forgiving each other.

Then Jesus was taken before the governmental

authorities of that day and eventually sentenced to death. He was mocked and beaten, a crown of thorns was pressed onto His head, and He was crucified on a cross. Jesus' sacrifice paid the penalty for our sin so that we can be brought back into relationship with Father God. Jesus said, *"I am the way and the truth and the life. No one comes to the Father except through Me." (John 14:6 NIV)*

Jesus took the punishment for my sin, for your sin, so that we can have ongoing fellowship with the Lord, with Father God. *"For God so loved the world that He gave His one and only Son, that whoever believes in Him shall not perish but have eternal life." (John 3:16 NIV)*

What makes His death different from all others? He did not stay in the grave. He conquered death, came back to life, rose on the third day, and is now with the Father. Jesus said, *"I am the resurrection and the life. The one who believes in me will live, even though they die." (John 11:25 NIV)*

But it does not stop there. Jesus is coming back to get His bride (those of us who believe in Him). Jesus said, *"Do not let your hearts be troubled. You believe in God, believe also in Me. My Father's house has many rooms; if that were not so, would I have told you that I am going there to prepare a place for you? And if I go and prepare a place for you, I will come back and take you to be with me that you also may be where I am." (John 14:1-3 NIV)*

In the meantime, He sent the Holy Spirit to empower us to do what we cannot do on our own … to live a righteous life. *"I will ask the Father, and he will give you another advocate to help you and be with you forever … the Advocate, the Holy Spirit, whom the Father will send in my* name, will teach you all things and will remind you of everything I have said to you." (John 14:16, 25-26 NIV)

Scripture tells us that he who believes **has** eternal life (John 5:24). That means that this relationship is for all time, even after our physical death. *"The gift of God is eternal life in Christ Jesus our Lord."* (Romans 6:23b NIV)

Would you like for God to walk with you through the mountains and valleys of this world, into eternity where there is no more disease, pain, sin? You can pray like this:

Father God, I am a sinner. I cannot save myself, but I believe that Jesus is Your Son and that He died to pay for my sin. He arose, conquering death once and for all, and He is now with You. I choose to follow You from this point forward. Teach me Your ways, Lord, and help me be obedient to Your will.

When you have surrendered your life to Christ, find a church family and get involved in the life of that church. Begin a daily study of scripture. Three options come to mind: the One Year Bible study, reading the gospels (Matthew, Mark, Luke, and John), or listening to scripture through a Bible app.

Talk to God throughout the day. There is no "right way" to pray. Just be yourself, tell Him your joys, sorrows, needs, wants. It may also help to follow the guiding steps of the Lord's Prayer *(Matthew 6:9-13).* It starts with praising God for who He is … Creator, Provider, Healer, Guide, Savior (there are even books about the names of God). Also remember what God says to be true about YOU! You are His treasure, you are loved, you have a purpose, He knows you intimately and cares about you.

Finally begin to share your faith with others. Your

testimony can inspire and encourage others on their own spiritual journeys. I am in a group of women whose children have special needs, Rising Above Ministries. On our difficult days, these women are God's light in the darkness. It's so easy to get stuck on our troubles but we start each meeting by sharing situations, items, events for which we are thankful. We call them "gratitudes." My friend of over forty years, Martha, was encouraged by God to start a blessing journal after her husband died suddenly and unexpectedly. What a blessing it is to share what another friend calls the "eye spy God" moments of our lives!

May God bless each of you with a closer walk with Father God and may He use you for His glory as you share life with others.

Conclusion

Information in this book is intended to challenge and encourage you to live a healthier life. I don't know if I have 20 minutes or 20 years to live, but I would like to live healthy.

As mentioned, a routine of exercise plus adequate amounts of sleep are not only critical for physical health but also for mental well-being. Even more important is daily time with Father God. Distraction is the devil's tool to redirect us, keep us busy and as far away from that relationship as possible. The Bible reminds us that *"God is our refuge and strength, an ever-present help in trouble. Therefore, we will not fear, though the earth give way and the mountains fall into the heart of the sea, though its waters roar and foam and the mountains quake with their surging. There is a river whose streams make glad the city of God, the holy place where the Most High dwells." (Psalm 46:1-4)* And guess what! We get to go there and live with Him forever if we have committed our lives to Christ.

Bob and I still try to maintain a mostly plant-based diet as suggested by Rip Esselstyn. However, we eat salmon once a week plus occasional chicken or venison. We also eat farm raised eggs from a trusted church friend for breakfast and in some recipes. As an alternative, you may replace eggs with Bob's Red Mill Egg Replacer, Simple Truth Organic Plant Based Egg Replacer, EnerG Egg Replacer or other similar products.

After learning about high density nutrients and lectins, I reviewed recipes in *Vegan Cuisine* and marked out items from Dr. Gundry's list of foods that have lectins. A few of those revised recipes plus new ones are included in this book. I have also added some recipes with high nutrient value according to lists provided in Dr. Fuhrman's book.

Notice that onions, sweet potatoes, and mushrooms are in many recipes because of their high nutritional value. Whatever you have done with white potatoes, you can do better with sweet potatoes. Cook chunks of sweet potatoes and mix with greens and onions. Make a loaded sweet potato with sour cream and chives (or broccoli and cheese). Use in Shepherd's Pie. You can also sprinkle Cinnamon Stevia over a buttered sweet potato or smother it with 100% Maple Syrup (recipes included). The dietician at a nearby assisted living suggested sprinkling sweet potato fries with nutmeg.

Although there are an increasing number of plant-based options in grocery stores (including Kroger's, Whole Foods, and Sprouts), be sure to lean towards fresh foods. Recipes included in this book should help you see how easy it is to incorporate healthy foods into your diet while deleting things that could damage your health. Also note that most of these recipes freeze well making it easier to double or triple your amount and freeze portions.

Speaking of frozen foods, if I were to suggest something for newlyweds or young people, my number one gift would be a small chest freezer. Why? Because it is a money saver, a time saver, and an emotional/physical relief!

My mother had a big freezer that was always loaded. In fact, we lived near the Gulf of Mexico and, when hurricanes blew through and electricity was shut down for several days to a week, our freezer full of food remained solid. (Warning: if it's NOT full, food will thaw more quickly).

I love sales! Because of my freezer, I can buy six big slabs of salmon (always check expiration dates) at half price and enjoy it over the next six weeks. ($36 saved!)

Because of my freezer, I purchase a month's worth of delicious homemade sourdough bread, burger buns, and even sourdough sweet rolls and freeze.

Create casseroles, soups, meatless loaves, in-season vegetables, and so on for two to four meals. After all, it takes no more time to prepare four meals than it does to make one (time and energy saver). Then, if you have had a busy day or do not feel like cooking, just pull a meal out of the freezer and warm it in the oven or microwave (an emotional and physical relief to this super busy wife, mother, nurse, and so on!)

Whether you prepare or purchase, remember my motto: EAT ONE, FREEZE ONE!

★★★★★★★★★★★★★★★★★★★★★

Now you know why the title of this book is _Introduction to Healthy Living: Recipes for Life._ There is obviously no way to cover all the facts, figures, and research presented by doctors and researchers from all over the world. In fact, there are often two views on any given topic (including lectins). This book is just an introduction. Hopefully, as you read, you will be inspired to develop a healthier, more intentional lifestyle spiritually ... physically ... emotionally and mentally ... and nutritionally.

APPETIZERS

CHICKEN-LESS SALAD DIP

1 package Jackfruit
2 Tbsp. Amish Wedding Southern Mild Chow-Chow (cauliflower-based relish)
Lemon Pepper and Garlic seasoning to taste
2-3 Tbsp. dairy free sour cream

Place Jack Fruit between paper towels and squeeze dry. Add remaining ingredients and process in blender until smooth. Add milk or water if dip is too thick. Serve with wheat free chips (Siete) or almond flour crackers.

CREAM CHEESE CELERY STUFFING
(from Vegan Cuisine by Vivian D. Cate)

1 package dairy free cream cheese
½ cup diced olives (green or black)
Onion juice (grate ½ onion)
½ cup chopped pecans or walnuts
2 Tbsp. plant-based mayonnaise

Pulse together in food processor. Add juice from the can of olives for extra moisture and flavor as needed. Stuff into two-inch slices of celery sticks.

FRUIT AND NUT ENERGY BARS
(from Vegan Cuisine by Vivian D. Cate)

1 cup dates
½ cup raisins
½ cup cranberries (optional: cherry flavored)
1 cup assortment of pecans or walnuts
2 tsp. almond extract
¼ cup water

Place all ingredients in food processor until blended. Press into medium size muffin tins. Freeze overnight; then carefully pry out of tins with dull knife and store in ziplock bag in your freezer.

SPINACH DIP
(from Vegan Cuisine by Vivian D. Cate)

1 cup Follow Your Heart or Simple Truth plant-based mayo
14 oz. container Tofutti or plant-based sour cream
1 pkg. Knorr vegetable recipe mix
16 oz. frozen, chopped spinach
(optional) 1 can water chestnuts or walnuts

Cook spinach, cool, and squeeze out liquids. Mix ingredients together and serve with vegetables. While this is delicious right away, the flavor permeates the dip and tastes much better the next day.

BEVERAGES

BOB'S THIRST-QUENCHING TEA
(from Vegan Cuisine by Vivian D. Cate)

2 green tea bags
8 cups water
1 cup Stevia
1/2 cup lemon juice (bottled)
8 cups cold
(optional) mint leaves

Boil 2 tea bags in 8 cups of water. Let tea steep over night or longer. Add Stevia and stir until dissolved. Add lemon juice (may use juice of 2 lemons) and cold water. Stir and store in refrigerator.

ALMOND JOY SMOOTHIE

1 scoop Gundry MD (chocolate) Proplant Complete Shake
½ cup grated coconut
½ cup frozen cherries (or ¼ c maraschino cherries with juice)
(optional: 1/2 tsp. almond extract)
1 cup water or almond milk

Proplant Complete Shake reportedly "supports muscle growth and recovery and it promotes smooth, comfortable digestion." Mix all ingredients in blender. May store in refrigerator for midmorning snack. *(see Suggested Resources for product information)*

NANO BANANA SMOOTHIE

2 bananas
2 scoops BioPharm Nano greens
2 scoops BioPharm Omegas
2 scoops BioPharm Protein
2-3 cups Almond or Coconut milk

BioPharm is another product we have used for over ten years with positive results. Place ingredients in blender and process. May store in refrigerator and serve as a midmorning or midafternoon snack. *(see Suggested Resources for product information)*

HOT SPICED TEA MIX
(from Vegan Cuisine by Vivian Cate)

2 cups instant tea (we prefer decaffeinated)
3 cups instant powdered lemonade
6-8 cups Stevia
2 tsp. cloves
2 tsp. cinnamon
2 tsp. nutmeg
4 cups instant powdered orange juice

Mix all ingredients and store in airtight containers. Fill a mug with hot spiced tea mix as a gift for someone.

BREADS

PLEADS

BOB'S WHEAT FREE BISCUITS

1 1/3 cup Cassava flour
2/3 cup Almond flour
4 tsp. baking powder
½ tsp. cream of tartar
½ tsp. sodium free salt (like Benson's)
1-2 Tbsp. Stevia
5 Tbsp. Earth Balance butter substitute
2/3-1 cup vanilla almond or coconut milk

Blend dry ingredients together. Cut butter substitute into flour mixture. Slowly add milk while blending. Roll out dough about 1 inch thick and cut into circles using a 2-inch biscuit cutter or glass. Bake in 450-degree oven for 10-12 minutes until brown.

BOB'S WHEAT FREE PANCAKES

¾ cup Cassava flour
¾ cup Almond flour
¾ cup Coconut flour
2 Tbsp. baking powder
½ cup Stevia
3 eggs
2 cups vanilla almond or coconut milk
4 Tbs virgin olive oil

Mix dry ingredients together, stir in milk and oil. Add extra milk if necessary. Pour batter into greased nonstick skillet and bake on medium heat until brown on the bottom. Flip and bake one more time (may use waffle machine).

SUGGESTION: Make your own biscuit or pancake mixes! Omitting milk, eggs, and butter, triple dry ingredients and freeze for later use.

CASSAVA BREAD

2 cups Cassava flour
1 tsp. baking powder
6 large eggs
1 tsp. salt (like sodium free Benson's)
1 tsp red wine vinegar
2 Tbsp. honey or maple syrup
1 cup Stevia
½ cup avocado or olive oil
½ cup water

Preheat oven to 350 degrees. Mix dry ingredients together. Mix liquids. Slowly add wet to dry while stirring. Pour batter into greased 9X5 loaf pan. Place in preheated oven for 1 hour. Remove and cool before cutting. Freezes well.

ALMOND FLOUR MUFFINS
(use as replacement for cornbread)

4 cups almond flour
1 cup flaxseed meal
8 eggs

2/3 cup almond milk
5 Tbsp olive oil
2 Tbsp. baking powder
2 cups Stevia

Mix ingredients and pour into muffin tins (2/3 full). Bake at 350 degrees until brown (about 30 minutes). Cool. Freeze muffins in ziplock bags. (Also makes 2 loaves of bread)

WHEAT FREE STUFFING
(altered from Joan's Turkey Stuffing)

1 box Thrive Market wheat free stuffing mix
(optional: 1 small loaf or 6-8 Almond flour muffins)
4 eggs or 4 tsp. egg replacer
1 large onion, diced
2 stalks chopped celery
Sage, lemon pepper to taste (Thrive Market mix already has seasoning)
1 large, grated apple
½ cup chopped pecans or walnuts
4 ounces diced mushrooms
Almond milk

Crumble muffins and add sage if not using Thrive Market's mix. Add remaining ingredients. Add enough milk to moisten mixture. Bake for 45-60 minutes at 350 degrees. Freezes well.

BREAKFASTS

MILLET FRUIT BOWL

1 cup cooked millet
Water
¼ coriander
2 bananas
1-2 chopped or grated apple
1 cup frozen blueberries
2 Tbsp. flaxseed meal
(optional) butter to taste

Cook millet per package instructions. Add remaining ingredients and stir. Add butter or honey as needed. (Bob makes a large batch of millet, and we freeze in smaller containers for later use.)

CHEESY MILLET

1 cup precooked millet
½ cup dairy free cheese
1 chopped onion
Lemon pepper to taste

Cook millet according to package instructions. Add cheese, onion, and lemon pepper and warm in microwave. Serves 2 people or half can be saved for another meal.

BOB'S SAUSAGE PATTIES

1 lb. of meatless crumbles
1 tsp. salt
2 tsp. ground sage
½ tsp. ground black pepper
½ tsp. dark brown sugar
¼ tsp. ground cloves
(optional) dash of red pepper
1 tsp. paprika
2/3 tsp. garlic powder
¼ tsp. marjoram
¼ tsp. thyme
¼ tsp. cumin
1 Tbsp. olive oil

Mix ingredients and form into patties. Cook in large skillet with olive oil.

CINNAMON FRUIT MILLET

1 cup precooked millet
1 tsp vanilla extract
¼ to ½ tsp. cinnamon
½ to ¾ cup blueberries or cherries
1 grated apples
1 Tbsp. flaxseed powder
¼ cup raisins
2 Tbsp. honey

Mix ingredients and warm in microwave or on stove.

SCRAMBLED EGGS WITH AVOCADO

4 eggs
½ cup dairy free cheese
1 Tbsp. olive oil
½ cup chopped onion
Lemon pepper to taste

Sautee onion in oil, blend with eggs and scramble. Add pepper and cheese, stir until cheese melts. Serve and eat with avocado.

DESSERTS

DESSERTS

HOMEMADE ICE CREAM
(from Vegan Cuisine by Vivian D. Cate)

2 cups So Delicious Vanilla Coconut Creamer
3 cups vanilla almond milk
½ cup sugar (or 1 cup Stevia)
Pinch of salt
Bag of crushed ice
Box of ice cream salt

Mix creamer, milk, sugar, and salt. Pour into ice cream freezer and add lid. Surround container with crushed ice and ice cream salt as per directions on freezer. Plug in and let it churn for about 30 minutes until the motor begins to slow down. Ice cream will be soft but, IF you don't eat it all first, it can go into your refrigerator freezer to harden!

ABSOLUTE BEST ICE CREAM SANDWICHES

Double chocolate wheat free cookie dough (homemade or from Thrive Market)
Dairy free ice cream (check local grocery stores or Thrive Market)

Bake cookies and freeze until cool. Meanwhile remove ice cream from freezer and allow to soften to consistency of mashed potatoes.

Place cooled cookies on flat surface (or use an extra-large glass container with lid). Cover each with ice cream topped with a second cookie. Return to freezer for a few hours. Enjoy!

WHEAT FREE PIE CRUST

1 cup almond flour
2 Tbsp. coconut flour
2/3 cup cassava flour
½ cup dairy free butter (or ghee)
¼-1/2 cup Stevia
1 large egg

Process the first 5 ingredients. Add egg and mix well into ball of dough. Roll out dough in a circle between 2 sheets of parchment paper. Place in pie pan and pierce dough 3-4 times with a fork. Partially bake crust at 375 degrees for 6-8 minutes until barely set (bake for 15 minutes for fully baked crust). Add ingredients for quiches, pot pies, or fruit pies and bake another 10 minutes.

WHEAT FREE CAKE

Duncan Hines KETO friendly yellow cake mix is made with almond and coconut flour. Nature's Eats Baking Genius also uses almond flour in their cake mix. These work well with all the cake recipes included in this book. There are wheat free recipes online.

STRAWBERRY SHORT CAKE

Wheat free cake mix (Duncan Hines, Nature's Eats, or homemade)
Reddi Whip Non-Dairy Vegan Whipped Topping (made with almond milk)
Sliced strawberries

Bake cake according to directions but add ½ cup chopped strawberries to cake mix before baking. Cool cake. Cover with whipped topping and decorate with sliced strawberries.

BANANA BLUEBERRY TRUFFLE

Wheat free cake mix (Duncan Hines, Nature's Eats, or homemade)
¾ cup frozen blueberries
1-2 sliced bananas
1 package banana pudding (mix according to directions)
¾-1 cup dairy free whipped cream

Bake cake according to package directions, cool, and then break baked cake into bite size pieces. Place ½ of each ingredient in large (preferably clear) bowl in order listed. Place other ½ of each ingredient on top. Serve and freeze leftovers for another meal.

CHOCOLATE CHERRY TRUFFLE

Wheat free cake mix (Duncan Hines, Nature's Eats, or homemade)
OR Duncan Heinz wheat free brownies baked
1 package chocolate pudding (mix according to directions)
1 small jar maraschino cherries
1 cup dairy free whipped cream (such as Reddi Whip Non-dairy whipped topping)
(optional: add 1 tsp. almond extract)

Bake cake or brownies according to package directions, cool, and then break into bite size pieces. Place ½ of each ingredient in large (preferably clear) bowl in order listed. Place other ½ of each ingredient on top. Serve and freeze leftovers for another meal.

FRUIT SALAD TRUFFLE

Wheat free cake mix (Duncan Hines, Nature's Eats, or homemade)
1 cup left over fruit salad
(Optional: Honey, walnuts, or pecans)
1 package vanilla pudding (mix according to directions)
1 cup dairy free whipped cream (such as Reddi Whip Non-dairy whipped topping)

Bake cake according to package directions, cool, and then break baked cake into bite size pieces. Follow instructions noted with previous truffles.

RYAN'S PINEAPPLE UPSIDE DOWN CAKE

1 box Duncan Hines wheat free cake mix or Nature's Eats
Baking Genius (almond flour cake mix)
2 eggs (or as per package instructions)
½ cup Earth Balance dairy free butter
1 ¼ cup water
2 tsp. almond extract
4 Tbsp. Earth Balance or dairy free butter
½ cup brown sugar
20 oz. can sliced pineapples (drained)
8 oz. jar maraschino cherries

Preheat oven to 350 degrees. Blend first five ingredients.
Set aside. Melt 4 Tbsp. butter with brown sugar in a
9X13 inch cake dish (do this in the oven). Place slices of
pineapple across bottom of cake dish on top of melted
butter and sugar. Put cherries in the center of each sliced
pineapple and pour batter over fruit. Bake for 30–35
minutes. Slightly cool; then turn cake over onto large
platter.

ENTREES

ENTRÉES

PARMESAN MUSHROOM CASSEROLE
(altered from Fungalicious recipe)

8 oz. sliced oyster mushrooms (fresh or Fungalicious)
2 cloves garlic or 2 tsp. garlic powder
1 large onion, chopped
2 Tbsp. olive oil
4 Tbsp. dairy free butter
1 cup Carrot juice (optional: water or vegetable broth)
1 tsp. lemon pepper
1 tsp. Mrs. Dash or other seasonings)
1 pkg. (8 oz.) frozen spinach or 2 cups fresh spinach
5-8 oz. grated Parmesan cheese
1 pkg. Palmini angel hair noodles or wheat free noodles

Sauté mushrooms, garlic, and onion in olive oil until onion is translucent. Add butter, onion, carrot juice, seasonings, and spinach. Cook on medium heat. Stir in grated parmesan cheese and serve over warmed noodles OR serve with almond flour muffins (homemade or Simple Mills Almond Flour Artisan Bread Mix).

MACARONI AND CHEESE

1 pkg. Palmini angel hair noodles
8 oz. dairy free cheese
2 Tbsp. dairy free butter
1 Tbsp. Cassava flour
¼ to ½ cup almond or coconut milk
2 tsp. garlic herbal seasoning (or Mrs. Dash Original)

Melt butter in saucepan. Blend in flour. Add cheese, milk, and seasonings, stirring until cheese melts and ingredients are smooth. Pour over warmed Palmini noodles and stir until they blend together.

VEGIE BEAN CHILI

1 cup dried red beans
1 cup dried black beans
1 cup dried pinto beans
3 cups water (or use vegetable stock from greens)
2 chopped onions
1 cup Fungalicious dried mushrooms (or 1 can mushrooms)
1 Tbsp. cumin
12oz. pkg frozen broccoli (or fresh broccoli)
12oz. pkg. frozen cauliflower (or fresh cauliflower)
3 cloves minced garlic (or garlic powder)
1pkg. taco seasoning

Pressure-cook beans with water as per pressure cooker instructions (cook until tender but not mushy). Sauté onions and mushrooms in olive oil. Add beans, broccoli, and cauliflower, and cook until vegetables are tender. Serve with wheat free chips or crackers or almond flour muffins.

WHITE BURGER ENCHILADAS

1 lb. plant-based meat
1 chopped onion

½ cup dehydrated Fungalicious Mushrooms (or 1 small can mushrooms)
4 Tbsp. dairy free butter
2 Tbsp. Cassava flour
1 cup almond or coconut milk
Benson's salt, pepper (or Mrs. Dash Lemon Pepper), and garlic
2 cups dairy free cheese (opt: dairy free sour cream to sauce)

Soften Fugalicious mushrooms in ¼ cup warm water. Sauté with meat and onions. Add ½ cheese. Place down the center of wheat free Siete or Sweet Potato tortillas and fold. Warm the butter, add flour and then milk while stirring. Warm until thick. Pour white sauce over enchiladas and top with rest of cheese. Bake at 350 degrees.

SWEET POTATO BLACK BEAN QUESADILLAS

1 medium sweet potato, grated
2 Tbsp. olive oil
1 tsp chili powder, ½ tsp cumin (optional: 1 pkg Taco seasoning and ¼ cup water)
8 grain free tortillas (8-10-inch diameter)
3 cups dairy free shredded cheddar or mozzarella cheese
1 cup pressure cooked black beans
2 tsp. avocado oil
1 chopped onion, sauteed
1 avocado, mashed
½ cup sour cream

Sauté chopped sweet potatoes and onion in olive oil. Add water and seasoning. Cook on medium heat until sweet potato is tender (about 10 minutes). Warm tortillas in skillet for about 30 seconds, flipping halfway through. Cover each of 4 tortillas with 1/3 cup of cheese, add ¼ of cooked sweet potato and onion, top with ¼ cup of beans. Sprinkle 1/3 cup cheese over fillings and cover each with an empty tortilla. Brush tops with light covering of olive oil and cook in skillet until edges brown, flip and cook until crispy. Blend avocado and sour cream into sauce and serve on top of each quesadilla. Option: Bob cooks tortillas on both sides and THEN adds warmed ingredients.

QUICK AND EASY QUESADILLAS

Follow the same instructions as above but spread each tortilla with mashed avocado, top with pressure cooked black beans or Dr. Praeger meatless patties, add dairy free Provolone cheese. Cook in skillet until edges brown.

CHIK-N-SALAD

1 package Jackfruit
2 Tbsp. Amish Wedding Southern Mild Chow-Chow (cauliflower- based relish)
2 sticks celery, chopped
Lemon Pepper and Garlic seasoning to taste
3-4 Tbsp. dairy free mayonnaise (such as Veganaise)

Place Jackfruit between 2 paper towels and press to dry. Add remaining ingredients. Makes a delicious sandwich or serve with wheat free chips (Siete) or almond flour crackers.

KIDNEY KALE KASSEROLE

1 pkg dried kidney beans
2 onions, diced
8 oz. mushrooms
1 Tsp. olive oil
12 oz. frozen kale (or 2-3 cups fresh kale)
Nondairy Parmesan cheese
¼ cup honey
½ cup brown sugar
¼ cup Bar B Q sauce

Pressure cook beans. Sauté onions and mushrooms in oil. Add kale, honey, brown sugar, and Bar B Q sauce to beans and vegetables. Warm and sprinkle with parmesan cheese.

PIZZA

½ cup almond flour
1/3 cup cassava flour
3 Tbsp ground flax seed (in 6 Tbsp. warm water)
1 tsp. baking powder
1 tsp. garlic powder
½ tsp. Italian seasoning
½ tsp. Benson Tasty Table (sodium free)

1 ½ Tbsp avocado oil
1 tsp. red wine vinegar

Mix ingredients into a ball, roll out into circle, and bake in a 400-degree oven for 10-12 minutes.

TOPPINGS

Instead of pizza sauce, spread Basil pesto or mashed avocado across pizza crust. Cover with chopped and/or grated vegetables (such as spinach or other greens, diced onions, mushrooms, cole slaw, chopped broccoli or cauliflower, grated carrots, artichokes). Be creative! You may also spread with meatless pepperoni, meat crumbles, or mushroom crumbles. Cover with dairy free cheese and sprinkle with basil. Bake another 10-12 minutes at 450 degrees.

MEATLESS LOAF

1 ½ lb. plant-based meat crumbles and/or mushroom crumbles
1 cup crushed wheat-free Taco chips, crackers or stuffing mix
2 eggs
Lemon pepper
2 Tbsp. liquid coconut amino's
3 Tbsp. honey mustard
3 Tbsp. brown sugar
1 chopped onion

½ cup mushrooms
1-2 stalks chopped celery
Garlic powder

Mix ingredients together. Mold and place in bread pan. May also form into small loaves (each for 2-3 persons) and bake on cookie sheets. Bake at 350 degrees for 1-1 ¼ hour. Freezes well!

SAUSAGE, KALE, AND WHITE BEAN STEW

1 pound white beans
2 cups kale
2 celery stalks, diced
1 cup grated carrots
2 onions, chopped
1 can mushrooms
1 pound plant-based smoked or kielbasa sausage
Lemon pepper to taste

Pressure-cook beans according to instructions. Mix with remaining ingredients, add water, and cook until vegetables are tender.

SWEET POTATO SHEPHERD'S PIE

2 large sweet potatoes
2 Tbsp. olive oil
1 large onion, diced

1 cup Fungalicious mushrooms (or 1 large can mushrooms)
2 cloves garlic, diced
Benson salt, lemon pepper
1 tsp coriander
1 tsp. oregano
1 tsp. basil
(optional: Taco seasoning)
1 lb. black beans, cooked in pressure cooker
2 8-ounce packages dairy free grated cheese
(optional: garnish with sour cream and diced avocado)

Microwave sweet potatoes for 7-10 minutes. Cut in half and remove pulp. Mash sweet potatoes and spread across bottom of 2 pie pans. Sauté onion, garlic, and mushrooms in oil. Add beans and seasoning. Pour over mashed sweet potatoes. Cover with cheese and melt in oven or microwave. Eat one, freeze one! This is one of our very favorite recipes, so I often make 3-4 pies at a time!

HICKORY SMOKED BEAN CASSEROLE

1 lb. beans (kidney or mixed)
½ cup coleslaw
2 large apples
2 small sweet potatoes
1 large onion
1 can mushrooms (or equivalent Fungalicious)
3-4 Tbsp. liquid smoke (to taste)
Lemon pepper and butter to taste

Pressure cook beans to remove lectins. Mix ingredients in crock pot, add water as needed, and cook on high until vegies are tender (3-4 hours) or on low overnight. Serve on Palmini or wheat free noodles.

CROCKPOT KALE AND BEANS

2 bunches fresh kale and/or spinach (2 bags frozen)
1 large onion, diced
8 oz. mushrooms, chopped (dried Fungalicious crumbled)
2-3 cloves garlic, minced
Lemon pepper and seasonings to taste
1 lb. dried black or red beans
Plant-based grated Parmesan cheese
Chopped walnuts

Pressure-cook beans to remove lectins. Pour all ingredients into crockpot and cook on high for 1-2 hours. Sprinkle Parmesan and walnuts over stew and serve.

SALADS

SWEET POTATO SALAD

2 sweet potatoes, cooked and cubed
½ cup Amish Wedding Southern Mild Chow-Chow (cauliflower-based relish)
1 Tbsp. mustard
3-4 Tbsp. Veganaise or plant-based mayonnaise
1 stalk celery, chopped
Mrs. Dash or Herb Garlic and Lemon Pepper to taste

Mix and mash ingredients together. Because cucumbers have lectins, we normally use Amish Wedding's cauliflower-based relish.

RED BEET COLE SLAW

1 pkg cole slaw mix
½ to ¾ cup canned beets, shredded
1 apple, grated
½ cup raisins
1/4 Red Wine or Balsamic vinegar
1/2 cup honey (or 2/3 cup Stevia)
1/2 cup Veganaise or other plant-based mayonnaise

Mix all ingredients and refrigerate for several hours or all night to enhance flavors.

MAMA MAVIS' LAYERED SALAD
(her original recipe used peas instead of broccoli)

Layer of lettuce (chopped into bite size pieces)
Layer of green onions (diced)
Layer of chopped celery
1 can sliced water chestnuts (or ½ cup walnuts)
Layer of fresh broccoli, chopped into bite size pieces
1 can mushrooms or 1 cup Fungalicious mushrooms
8 ounces Veganaise or other dairy free dressing
1 package dairy free grated cheddar cheese

Layer ingredients as noted. Soften Fungalicious mushrooms in ½ cup warm water and drain before placing on top of broccoli. Cover salad with another layer of lettuce. Then spread jar of dressing across the top like icing. Sprinkle with 1 package cheese and refrigerate 8-10 hours. (Optional: mix dressing with dairy free sour cream; season plant-based bacon with garlic, fry in skillet, crumble and sprinkle on top)

PASTA BROCCOLI CARROT SALAD

1 cup Jovial grain-free cassava Fusilli or Palmini noodles
1 cup Broccoli, chopped into bitesize pieces
1 cup Carrots, finely chopped or grated
½ cup Green or black onions, diced
½ cup honey
½ cup olive oil
½ cup Balsamic or Red Wine vinegar

Cook pasta. Mix with vegetables and sauce. Refrigerate overnight.

TACO CHIP BEAN SALAD
(adapted from Mama Mavis' recipe)

1 large can Ranch Style beans, drained
1 bottle Italian Wishbone dressing
1 head of lettuce (or mixture of greens)
3 green onions
Lemon pepper, garlic powder, herbal seasoning (Mrs. Dash)
1 lb. meatless crumbles (optional: mushroom crumbles)
1 cup grated dairy free cheese

Marinate beans in Italian dressing overnight. Shred lettuce 1chop green onions and toss with seasonings over lettuce/greens. Brown meatless crumbles according to package directions and cover salad. Top with marinated beans and Italian dressing (do not drain). Cover with cheese and serve with wheat free taco chips or crackers.

FRUIT SALAD

1 pear, cut in bite size pieces
1 banana, sliced
1 peach, cut in bite size pieces
1 mango, cut in bit size pieces
Walnuts or pecans, chopped
Raisins or grapes
Dried cranberries

Honey

Mix seasonal fruit of any kind. Add remaining ingredients plus honey to taste. Freezes well so double or triple amount.

MAMMA JOAN'S BROCCOLI SALAD

1 head of broccoli, cut into bite size pieces
1 pkg. dairy free cheddar cheese, grated or cut in bite size chunks
½ to 1 finely diced onion
½ to ¾ cups dried cranberries and raisins
3-4 Tbs. dairy free mayonnaise

Mix and put in the refrigerator overnight.

THREE BEAN SALAD

½ cup dried kidney beans
½ cup dried white or Northern beans
½ cup dried pinto beans
1 large onion, chopped
1/2 olive oil
1/2 cup red wine vinegar
1 cup Stevia

Cook beans according to pressure cooker directions. Mix olive oil, vinegar, and Stevia. Add chopped onions and stir into bean mixture. Store overnight in the refrigerator (so that flavors are absorbed into the beans).

SANDWICHES

SANDWICHES

BANANA BUTTER OPEN FACE

2 slices wheat free or sourdough bread
4 Tbsp. almond butter
1 banana, sliced lengthwise

Toast bread in air fryer or broil in oven. Spread each slice with almond butter and cover with sliced banana. Serve with Sweet Potato Soup.

JACKFRUIT SALAD SANDWICH

1 pkg. Jackfruit
1 stalk celery, chopped
2 Tbsp. Amish Wedding Southern Mild Chow-Chow (cauliflower-based relish)
Veganaise or other dairy free dressing
Lemon pepper and Herb garlic seasoning to taste
4 slices wheat free or sourdough bread

Mix and spread large amount on bread, cover with second slice of bread. Serve with a cup of hot soup.

GRILLED JACKFRUIT SANDWICH

Add ½ cup grated carrots and ¼ cup diced onion. Spread mixture on one slice of bread, cover with a slice of dairy free cheese, and top with second slice of bread. Butter the outer sides of sandwich, brown in skillet until brown, turn sandwich over and repeat grilling process.

BLOC SANDWICH
Bacon, Lettuce, Onion, Cheese

2 slices sourdough or wheat free bread
2 slices plant-based bacon (Lightlife Smart Bacon)
Garlic powder to taste
1 slice onion
1 large leaf lettuce
Dairy free mayonnaise (like Veganaise)
Slice of dairy-free smoked, cheddar, or provolone cheese

Sprinkle each bacon strip with garlic. Fry bacon in skillet with dab of olive oil. Toast bread in air fryer or oven. Spread each piece with mayonnaise. Layer bacon, onion, lettuce, and cheese on one slice and cover with the other. Enjoy while hot!

LOADED BURGERS

2 slices Cassava or sourdough bread, toasted
Veganaise and mustard
Slice of onion
Slice of dairy free cheese
½ onion, chopped
5-7 mushrooms (or hydrated Fungalicious mushrooms)
1 Dr. Praeger plant-based burger
1 Tbsp. olive oil

Sautee chopped onion and mushrooms in oil. Cook burger according to package directions. Spread each slice of toast with Veganaise and mustard. Layer toast with burger, onion slice, cheese, sauteed vegetables. Cover with second toast or serve open faced.

GRILLED CHEESE SANDWICH

2 slices almond or sourdough bread
1-2 slices dairy free smoked cheddar or provolone cheese
Veganaise and mustard
2 Tbsp. dairy free butter
(optional: sprinkle with Basil)

Spread Veganaise and mustard on bread. Fill with cheese and close the sandwich. Butter the outsides of sandwich, grill on skillet until brown, turn over and repeat the grilling process.

OPEN FACE AVOCADO SANDWICH

Spread sourdough bread with Veganaise, top with thick slices sliced avocado (optional: add dairy free cheese). Season with lemon pepper.

EMPANADAS

Wheat free biscuit dough
Jackfruit salad OR cheese and Tofurky hickory smoked deli slices
Veganaise and mustard to taste

Roll out dough and cut into 4 large round circles (may use sandwich plate as pattern to cut around). Spread each with plant-based dressing and mustard. Fill the center with salad or cheese and sandwich slices. Fold in half and seal edges with fork all around. Bake in oven at 350 degrees until brown, turn over and bake until brown.

SOUPS

SWEET POTATO SOUP

4 cups apple cider or water
1 large onion, chopped
2 large sweet potatoes, skin removed
2 large apples, with or without skins
2 tsp. coriander
2 tsp. ginger
3 garlic cloves, minced or 2 tsp. garlic powder
1-2 cups almond or coconut milk

Cube sweet potato skin. Cut apples into large chunks. Mix all ingredients soft (on high for several hours or on low overnight). Puree in blender, add milk to preferred consistency.

BASIL CORIANDER VEGIE BEAN SOUP

1 bottle carrot juice
1 pkg. cole slaw
1 pkg. mixed greens
1 cup water
1cup mushrooms
1 chopped onion
1 pkg dried beans, pressure cooked
2 Tbs each of basil and oregano
2 tsp. each of coriander and cumin
Lemon pepper or Bensons Tasty Table
6 Tbsp. red wine vinegar

Cook in a crockpot on high until tender. Puree 2 cups of stock in blender and return to pot of soup to thicken.

VEGETABLE BEAN SOUP

3 Tbsp. olive oil
6 stalks celery, diced
2 large carrots, diced or grated
1 large onion, chopped
8 oz. can mushrooms (or hydrated Fungalicious mushrooms)
2 lb. broccoli
5 cups water
2 Tbsp. Cassava flour
1 ½ cups almond or coconut milk
Lemon Pepper and Mrs. Dash (or other seasonings to taste)

Sauté celery, carrots, onion, and mushrooms in oil until soft. Pressure-cook dried beans to remove lectins. Mix sautéed vegetables and beans with water and broccoli. Cook until broccoli is tender. Remove ½ broth and stir slowly into flour until smooth. Add milk while stirring. Then mix back into soup.

We do not care for watery soup. Two methods of thickening are noted in this recipe and in the following Vegie Lentil Soup recipe.

VEGIE LENTIL SOUP

4 cups carrot juice

3-4 cups water

6-8 bag cole slaw

4 cups fresh or frozen spinach

1 chopped onion

2 chopped carrots

2 stalks celery, diced

1 lb. bag dried lentils

1 sweet potato, chopped into bitesize pieces

1 cup Stevia

1 Tbsp. oregano

2 tsp. basil

1 tsp. ground coriander

1 tsp. cumin

Lemon pepper

6 cups water

(optional: ¼ tsp. liquid smoke)

Place ingredients in a crockpot and cook on high for 4-6 hours. Pour 2 cups of soup (with liquids) into blender and puree. Add mixture back into soup.

Note that carrot juice can be used in place of water or vegetable broth for a thicker and more delicious soup.

BROCCOLI CHEESE SOUP
(adapted from Vegan Cuisine by Vivian D. Cate)

3-4 stalks celery, chopped
1 onion, diced
1 cup carrots, grated
4-6 ounces mushrooms, diced (or Fungalicious mushrooms)
1 large head of broccoli (or package of broccoli florets)
2 cups carrot juice (or 1 package vegetable broth)
1-2 cups water
1 cup almond or coconut milk
1 cup grated dairy free cheese

Mix ingredients except for milk and cook on high in crockpot for 3 to 4 hours (or on low over night). Remove 1/3 to ½ of soup, add milk, and puree. Return to main pot of soup and blend.

MUSHROOM SOUP

2 Tbsp dairy free butter
2 Tbsp cassava flour
1 ¼ cup almond milk
1 can mushrooms (or equivalent Fungalicious)

Sautee mushrooms in a tablespoon of olive oil. Melt butter, blend in flour while stirring. Add milk and continue to stir (over heat) until thick. Stir in mushrooms.

NOTE: Cassava is an edible tuber or root vegetable, sometimes known as yuca. The flour has thickening ability similar to whole wheat or white flour so it is often used in plant-based foods.

VEGETABLES

LOADED SWEET POTATOES

1 medium sweet potato
2 Tsp. sour cream
1 Tbsp. chives
(optional: steamed broccoli, ½ cup grated dairy free cheese)

Bake potato for 8-10 minutes in microwave. Cut in half and remove skin. Mash and top with sour cream and chives. (Makes a delicious breakfast!)

BOB'S MAPLE SYRUP
SWEET POTATOES

Cook sweet potato in microwave for 8-10 minutes depending on size. Mash and add maple syrup to taste.

CAULIFLOWER MASH

Cook cauliflower until tender. Add seasonings and puree in a blender. Serve as a healthy replacement for mashed Irish potatoes.

GRILLED OR ROASTED VEGETABLES

Carrots and/or brussels sprouts
Broccoli and/or cauliflower
Sweet potatoes
Olive Oil

Drench vegetables with olive oil and roast at 400 degrees, turning every 10 minutes until tender. (Optional: toss with dairy free Parmesan, garlic, herbs, or lemon pepper as desired).

BOB'S MARINATED VEGIE SNACKS

Cook carrots, cauliflower, broccoli florets, or other vegetables until mildly tender. Pour a mixture of 1/3 olive oil, 1/3 cup red wine vinegar, and 1/3 honey over vegetables. Store in refrigerator for 24 hours to allow vegetables to absorb flavors.

JOAN'S MARINATED CARROTS
(from Vegan Cuisine by Vivian Cate)

2 lb. carrots (boil until soft)
1 medium onion, chopped
¾ cup vinegar
1 tsp. prepared mustard
1 tsp. salt free liquid coconut aminos
1 ½ cups Stevia
¼ cup olive oil

Mix ingredients and store in refrigerator for 24 hours to absorb flavors.

VEGETABLE POT PIE

1 wheat free pie crust
Handful of greens
1 small package frozen broccoli
1 sweet potato skinned and cut in bitesize pieces
1 can mushrooms
1 onion
1 Tbsp cassava flour
1 Tbsp. dairy free butter
1 cup almond or coconut milk
1 cup dairy free grated cheese
Season to taste
(optional: use a mixture of leftover cooked vegetables)

Cook vegetables until tender. Add flour to melted butter, stirring continually. Add milk and cook until thickened. Blend vegetables with white sauce and cheese. Bake pie crust in 350 degree oven for 5-7 minutes (remove when it starts to brown). Pour vegetable mixture into pie crust and bake until edges of crust are dark brown.

Optional: serve vegetable/white sauce blend over wheat free noodles instead of in a pie crust.

COOKED GREENS

How do we cook greens when we are not supposed to eat pork or bacon? Here's an option: cut a sweet potato into bite size pieces. Chop one or two onions plus some mushrooms. Mix with assorted greens and cook in crockpot until tender. This is also good with Bob's sauce of 1/3 vinegar, 1/3 olive oil, and 1/3 honey. Make enough to freeze a few portions for later.

STIR FRY

Salad (a great way to use up leftovers!)
Greens
Cole Slaw (without sauce)
Onions and mushrooms
Broccoli, chopped or riced
Cauliflower, chopped or riced
Herbs, garlic, Mrs. Dash original, Benson's Table Tasty
Liquid Amino's

Pour ¼ cup olive oil into large skillet. Add vegetables as desired (add more olive oil as needed). Add seasonings and liquid amino's to taste. Serve over cooked millet, as a side dish, or freeze portions for later.

SWEET POTATO CASSEROLE

2 lb. bag of Alexis (or other brand) sweet potato puffs
¼ cup dairy free butter (such as Earth Balance)
1 can mushroom soup (or see recipe for Mushroom Soup)
1 chopped onion
1 pint dairy free sour cream
1 ½ cup grated dairy free cheddar cheese
(optional: 1 cup frosted flakes and ½ cup dairy free butter)

Defrost potato puffs. Mix with melted butter, mushroom soup, onion, sour cream and cheese. Place in container and bake 30 minutes at 350 degrees. Top with mixture of melted butter and frosted flakes and bake another 10–15 minutes.

NON-VEGAN, LECTIN FREE

BAKED CHICKEN

¼ cup brown sugar
½ tsp. garlic powder
½ tsp. lemon pepper
1 tsp basil
2 tsp Italian seasoning
4 chicken thighs
4 Tbsp. olive oil

Mix ingredients and pour over chicken. Bake at 425 degrees for 30 minutes until chicken is browned throughout.

ITALIAN SEASONED CHICKEN

Pour a bottle of Zesty Italian Dressing over 8 chicken thighs and marinate overnight. Grill or bake in oven at 350 degrees for 45 minutes. Delicious! Freeze to have on hand when you want to take a meal to someone.

LEMON SALMON

An easy way to cook slabs of salmon is to place in cake dish, pour about ½ cup lemon juice over the meat, season heavily with lemon pepper and bake at 350 degrees for 20 to 30 minutes or until no longer pink in the middle. This pairs well with asparagus and mandarin oranges.

VENISON STEW

Our son enjoys hunting with his friend. Every year he brings home a deer, and we pay to have it processed. The meat, however, is tough so we put it in a crockpot with cubed sweet potatoes, carrots, onions, and mushrooms. Add seasonings such as Lemon Pepper and Mrs. Dash or Herbal Garlic seasoning. Fill crockpot with 3 to 4 cups of water and cook all day or overnight on low until meat falls apart with a fork. Serve with a fruit salad.

SALMON CROQUETTES

1 can salmon (or fresh)
2 eggs
½ cup wheat free chips or crackers, crushed
1 stalk celery, diced
1 onion, chopped
Seasoning (such as Mrs. Dash, lemon pepper)

Mix and mold into patties, oil skillet and fry croquettes until brown on each side. Serve with Honey Mustard dressing: 1/3 honey, 1/3 mustard, 1/3 Veganaise.

CURRIED CHICKEN AND GREENS

1 large can chicken (may use a package of Jackfruit)
½ cup mushrooms, diced
1 medium onion, chopped
1 Tbsp. olive oil

1 pkg frozen spinach (or other greens)
Curry to taste
Dairy free parmesan cheese

Sauté mushrooms and onions in oil. Mix ingredients together and heat. Serve over wheat free noodles and sprinkle with parmesan cheese.

ORIENTAL CHICKEN

6 oz. skinless, boneless chicken breast
2 lb. broccoli florets (fresh or frozen)
½ walnuts, pecans, or almonds
6 oz. can mushrooms (or use fresh)
1 onion, chopped
20 oz. can pineapple (save juice)
2 Tbsp. cassava flour
¼ cup Stevia
1 Tbsp. Bragg's Liquid Aminos

Steam the chicken and broccoli for about 25 minutes. Dice into small chunks. Add mushrooms and nuts, pineapple chunks, Stevia, and liquid aminos. Add pineapple juice slowly (while stirring) to flour and simmer for 2 to 3 minutes until thickened. Add remaining ingredients. Freezes well.

JOANNIE'S CASSEROLE

We lived near the Gulf of Mexico where my mother, to whom this book is dedicated, used to purchase 100 pounds of shrimp from local shrimpers at 85 cents/pound. She then froze the meat in empty milk cartons. Mother purchased another 100 pounds for her sister who drove from Pennsylvania and packed it in dry ice for her return home. This was my favorite of mother's shrimp recipes. However, as previously mentioned, shrimp are scavengers and not a healthy choice. Supplement with chicken or fish.

1 Tbsp. cassava flour
2 cups almond milk
2 Tbsp. dairy free butter
2 to 3 cups fresh spinach (may use frozen spinach)
mushrooms and onions (sautéed)
2 to 3 Tbsp nutmeg (to taste)
Chicken or fish

Make white sauce by melting butter and adding flour while stirring. Add milk (continue to stir) and warm until thickened. Sauté mushrooms and onions and add to sauce. Pour over cooked chicken or fish. Season with nutmeg and serve over wheat free (such as Cabella's Fettuccini) or Palmini noodles

Resources

FORKS OVER KNIVES (a video with information from T. Colin Campbell, PhD and Caldwell Esselstyn, Jr. MD) www.forksoverknives.com

THE ENGINE 2 DIET by Rip Esselstyn
ISBN 978-0-446-50669-4
Published by Wellness Central, Hachette Book Group, New York/Boston

THE CHINA STUDY by T. Colin Campbell, PhD and Thomas M. Campbell, II. Published by BenBella Books, Dallas, Texas. ISBN978-1-932100-66-2

WHAT THE BIBLE SAYS ABOUT HEALTHY LIVING by Rex Russell, M.D. Published by Fleming H. Revell, a division of Baker Book House Co., Grand Rapids, Michigan.

3 STEPS TO INCREDIBLE HEALTH by Joel Fuhrman, MD
ISBN 978-0-9799667-8-1
Published by Gift of Health Press, Flemington, New Jersey

THE LONGEVITY PARADOX by Steven R. Gundry, MD
ISBN 978-0-06-284339-5
Published by HarperCollins Publishers, New York, NY

NanoGreens, NanoReds, NanOmega, NanoPro, and EPA pockets are researched, developed, and distributed by BioPharma Scientific, Inc., San Diego, CA 92121; for information go to www.superfoodsolution.com (products must be ordered from a licensed medical professional).

FUNGALICIOUS GOURMET MUSHROOMS
Naturally Grown since 2016, sustainably farmed
Tullahoma, Tennessee 37388
931-408-0382 or fungalicious.net
(they have several types of dried mushrooms, ask about mail orders)

SOURDOUGH BREAD SOURCES
Krogers and other local grocery stores have sourdough bread. If you live near an Amish or Mennonite community, you may also have access to sourdough bread. In the Winchester, Tennessee area we are blessed to have:

Swiss Pantry,
10026 David Crockett Hwy,
Belvidere, Tn 37306 (931-962-0567)

We also have a source in the Winchester Tennessee area, a lady who not only makes sourdough bread and burger buns but also the most delicious sourdough sweet rolls we have ever tasted!

Please note, you are encouraged to do your own research on information shared as well as for any products that may be listed or sold by persons mentioned in this book. Also speak with your doctors regarding changes in your diet. This book is an INTRODUCTION to get you thinking about living a healthier and happier life!

Printed in the United States
by Baker & Taylor Publisher Services

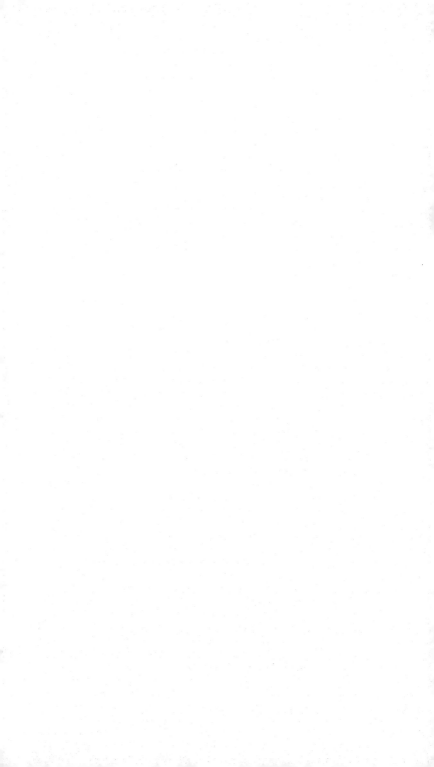